Clean Eating

Exquisite Culinary Creations For Enhancing Vitality,
Attaining Optimal Well-Being, And Realizing The
Aspired State Of Health And Wellness

(Boost Your Energy Levels And Facilitate Weight Loss)

Franklyn Proctor

TABLE OF CONTENT

The Tenets Of Nutrient-Rich Consumption................. 1

What Is Clean Eating?..14

The Rise And Notion Of Dietary Cleanliness............31

Benefits Of Clean Eating....................................46

Meal Planning And Recipes................................60

Health Benefits...74

Engage In Smart Meal Preparation And Consider Healthier Eating Options....................................79

Utilize The Principles Of Clean Eating To Benefit Your Health..99

Exploring The Relationship Between Metabolism And Clean Eating..128

Cherry Tomato Soup..152

Directions:...153

Paleo Egg Muffin Recipe 156

Grilled Chicken Panzanella 160

Spicy Miso And Pumpkin Soup 164

The Tenets Of Nutrient-Rich Consumption

The practice of clean eating extends beyond mere dietary choices; it is ingrained in one's lifestyle. Consuming unprocessed, nutrient-rich, and wholesome meals, combined with suitable physical activity, has the potential to enable individuals to live a highly healthful and prosperous life henceforth.

I would like to inform you that there is always an opportunity to amend the behaviors that are not contributing to the realization of your envisioned goals and aspirations. For a prolonged duration, I endured various detrimental and deleterious dietary regimens prior to acquiring the knowledge of consuming nourishment appropriately. The crucial aspect is that I managed to alleviate all the symptoms I had been experiencing due to an unhealthy lifestyle by adopting a nutritious diet and regular physical activity.

Embracing and adhering to a wholesome dietary regimen proves to be significantly more effortless than the majority of individuals perceive. If you conscientiously bear in mind the subsequent principles, maintaining adherence to a clean eating regimen should prove notably uncomplicated.

They are as follows:

It is advised to limit or, if possible, eradicate your consumption of processed foods.

When engaging in the act of shopping, it is advisable to consistently prioritize the selection of fresh, unprocessed, and unadulterated food items rather than opting for ones enclosed in packaging such as boxes, cans, or bags. Processed food products typically contain substantial quantities of various artificial additives and preservatives. The consumption of excessive amounts of these chemicals and preservatives can contribute to the development of numerous health issues in the future. Therefore, it is imperative to prioritize the consumption of predominantly fresh and organic foods if one desires to maintain good health in the long run.

Elevate your consumption of unprocessed carbohydrates.

Several excellent options comprise legumes, beans, and whole grains, such as brown rice, amaranth, millet, and quinoa. Sweeteners such as honey, agave nectar, and maple syrup can also be utilized sparingly as alternatives to granulated sugar.

It is imperative that each meal incorporates an appropriate balance of proteins, fats, and carbohydrates to promote overall health.

A balanced diet is crucial in staying healthy. "Ensure that your daily dietary intake incorporates a substantial yet balanced proportion of proteins, fats, and carbohydrates." I would like to refrain from adding unnecessary complexity, thus I will keep it uncomplicated in order to assist you in initiating the process.

A number of fantastic sources that are high in protein include chicken, turkey, salmon, extra lean ground beef, flank steak, tofu, tempeh, cottage cheese, and Greek yogurt.

Some exceptional sources of carbohydrates that promote a nutritious way of living encompass brown rice (which I incorporate into my daily diet), russet potatoes, sweet potatoes, oatmeal, quinoa, and lentils. Numerous fruits and vegetables exhibit a considerable carbohydrate content as well. In addition to furnishing vital micronutrients, fruits and vegetables possess the remarkable attribute of being low in calories, thereby enabling you to indulge in an ample quantity of them without incurring undesired weight gain. Consuming vegetables rich in dietary fiber facilitates enhanced waste elimination in the body, promoting greater efficacy and efficiency, thereby potentially aiding in weight reduction. A selection of excellent fruits and vegetables comprises blueberries, raspberries, strawberries, apples, bananas, oranges, tomatoes, kale, spinach, broccoli, brussel sprouts, carrots, and bell peppers.

In conclusion, several imperative sources of high fat in one's diet encompass eggs (including the yolk), almonds, walnuts, avocados, coconut oil, olive oil, a wide selection of cheeses, and even dark chocolate (which serves as an excellent alternative to milk chocolate, cake, and cookies...in addition, it possesses antioxidant properties!)

Exercise caution when consuming excessive amounts of salt, sugar, and fat.

Processed foods typically exhibit high caloric density, characterized by a substantial concentration of calories; additionally, they tend to possess elevated levels of sodium, glucose, and lipids. Once you have restricted or eliminated the consumption of processed foods from your dietary intake, you will encounter increased difficulty in maintaining your current level of daily caloric intake. Due to the reduction of calorie intake, your body will initiate the utilization of stored fat as a source of energy, facilitating weight loss as a result.

Before we proceed, I would like to provide further clarification regarding my previous mention to exercise caution with respect to fats. The aforementioned essential fats, despite being highly nutritious, possess a considerable caloric content. Each gram of fat is comprised of 9 calories, while each gram of protein and carbohydrates consists of 4 calories (it is worth noting that alcohol provides 7 calories per gram).

It is imperative to incorporate these fats into your diet; however, exercise caution and refrain from excessive consumption. To illustrate, it is quite astounding to witness the unexpectedly high caloric content present in a portion of nuts. If you have hitherto overlooked or lacked awareness regarding your dietary intake, I would highly recommend procuring a food scale and diligently employing it for approximately one week, thereby acquiring a more accurate comprehension of the caloric content you consume.

Refrain from consuming beverages with a high caloric content.

Carbonated beverages, fruit-based beverages, and alcoholic beverages all possess an overwhelmingly substantial caloric content. The habitual intake of these beverages has the potential to lead to a surplus of calories, consequently rendering weight loss exceedingly difficult. Furthermore, it is paramount to acknowledge that these products are detrimental to one's overall health. I would like to emphasize that I am not advocating for complete abstinence from these drinks, as I hold the belief that moderation is key. However, I strongly suggest restricting the intake of these beverages to a maximum frequency of twice weekly. It is recommended to primarily opt for water (90% of the time), coffee, and tea as they are more advantageous in enhancing overall well-being. In addition, it is worth noting that all of them possess a caloric content of zero.

Exercise

It is imperative to engage in physical activity if one desires weight loss and seeks to attain a long, healthy, and prosperous existence. Furthermore, engaging in consistent physical activity can effectively enhance the strength of your musculoskeletal system, thereby effectively mitigating the risk of enduring chronic injuries as you progress through the aging process. Based on your present state of health, mobility, and physical fitness, I advise incorporating a combination of high-intensity intervals of cardiovascular exercise, such as sprints, along with longer intervals of lower-intensity cardio activities like brisk walking or gentle jogging. Additionally, incorporating resistance training, which encompasses weightlifting and strength exercises, is essential for fostering muscle growth and mitigating the risk of injuries. Nevertheless, this suggestion pertains solely to individuals of average health and should be taken into consideration. I would suggest engaging the services of an individual who possesses the ability to tailor a fitness program specifically designed to cater to your unique requirements.

What Is Clean Eating?

The concept of clean eating entails consuming foods in their most unprocessed and natural form achievable. This refers to food products devoid of any synthetic colorings, flavorings, or preservatives. It also entails refraining from consuming excessively processed or refined foods, those containing refined sugar and bleached flour. Moreover, it involves abstaining from fried food and beverages laden with high amounts of sugar. Essentially, you consume the foods that our bodies have gradually adapted to consume and metabolize.

The concept of clean eating does not strictly conform to the definition of a diet. It pertains to a way of living. This is not a transient endeavor that one undertakes for a brief period and then reverts to consuming processed, artificial sustenance. After adhering to a clean diet for an extended period, it is possible that you may discover these particular foods to be gastric irritants. Furthermore, it should be noted that clean eating does not encompass the act of depriving oneself. It revolves around the selection of more intelligent dietary options. There exists a plethora of excellent clean eating recipes that possess remarkable flavor simultaneously. One can even engage in the process of cookie production.

A useful method to ascertain the cleanliness of a food product lies in establishing whether it has been tampered with by individuals. This implies enhancing the flavor, appearance, durability, and other characteristics by incorporating additional components. It is desirable for food to retain its natural state as much as possible. When food undergoes modification through the addition of chemicals, coloring agents, and similar substances, its nutritional value becomes diminished. Nutritious food is characterized by its minimal levels of sodium, fat, sugar, and artificial substances. If the packaging contains any components in the list of ingredients that possess characteristics resembling those of a scientific undertaking, it can be inferred that the food product does not adhere to cleanliness standards. The most sanitary food options are organic fruits and vegetables, however, there are alternative choices available to you.

There are numerous advantages associated with consuming healthy, unprocessed foods. Not only will it aid in combatting or preventing various illnesses, but it will also enhance your level of energy. Moreover, you will be capable of effectively managing stress and maintaining emotional stability. It enhances your metabolism, thus aiding in sustainable weight loss.

The clean diet is a highly effective approach for individuals seeking weight loss. As you are providing your body with the nutrients it is naturally meant to utilize, it will respond by initiating weight loss if necessary. Part of eating clean also means not counting calories or feeling hungry.You eat small clean meals frequently to keep your metabolism revved up and combine a lean protein, complex carb and healthy fat into every meal. In addition, your body will function more efficiently as it will not have to contend with the various chemicals present in processed food.

Embracing a clean eating lifestyle may require a change in mindset, but it can be easily implemented. The outcomes are prompt, and you will experience an almost immediate improvement in your well-being. Additionally, one will come to comprehend the multitude of chemicals that permeate our bodies by means of the sustenance we consume orally. It is quite daunting when one comes to that understanding.

What is the concept of clean eating and the permissible food selections?

Maintaining or achieving weight loss can be effectively accomplished through the practice of clean eating. However, what precisely constitutes clean eating or the permissible foods within a clean eating regimen. Clean eating involves consuming foods in their most natural state. Therefore, we do not offer processed, prepackaged meals that contain additional preservatives, sweeteners, and sodium. Essentially, if an object retains its original form as created by a divine being, it is considered to be pure.

Below is a comprehensive compilation to assist you in initiating a clean eating regimen.

Complex carbohydrates with high starch content

Consume a daily diet consisting of two to four servings of complex carbohydrates derived from starchy carbohydrate sources or whole grains.

The recommended portion for each of these items equates to the volume contained within a cupped hand.

Whole Grains

Vegetable Sources

Buckwheat

Bananas

Varieties of bread and wraps available include multi-grain, buckwheat, Ezekiel, oat bran, and whole-meal spelt.

Carrots

Oat-bran cereal

Potatoes

Oatmeal

Radishes

Quinoa

Sweet Potatoes

Spelt

Yams

Whole Barley

Chickpeas (Garbanzo beans)

Whole-wheat or brown rice couscous" can be rephrased in a formal tone as: "Couscous made from whole wheat or brown rice

Kidney beans

Whole-wheat, brown-rice, or other pasta made from whole grains.

Lentils

Unrefined, ebony or chestnut-colored rice

Navy beans

Pinto beans

Soybeans (edamame)

Split peas

Protein

Strive to consume a minimum of five to six servings of protein per day.

A suitable amount of protein corresponds to the dimensions of an individual's palm.

The protein consumed should originate from sources of lean meats, poultry, fish and eggs, dairy products, as well as select vegetable and grain sources.

Lean meats such as chicken and bison, as well as poultry and fish.

Eggs

Dairy

Tofu, chia seeds (also known as Salba), quinoa, and hemp seeds (offering a vegan alternative)

Dry beans that have been purchased and prepared manually (suitable for a vegan diet).

Nuts, Seeds, and Nut Butters (vegan alternative)

Contain a significant quantity of protein but a considerable amount of fat. While this fat is nutritious, it is advisable to moderate its consumption. Serving: Consume a single small handful of nuts or two tablespoons of nut butter daily.

Dietary Carbohydrates Derived from Fruits and Vegetables

A suitable quantity of fruits and vegetables consists of four to six servings of fresh produce per day.

The recommended portion size for fruits and vegetables is equivalent to two cupped hands.

Complex Carbohydrates Derived from Fruit

Artichokes

Apples

Asparagus

Berries

Beet Greens

Consuming dried fruits in moderation "Dried fruits in a balanced quantity"

"Eating dried fruits moderately" "In a measured amount, dried fruits"

Broccoli

Grapefruit

Brussels sprouts

Grapes

Cabbage

Kiwi

Cauliflower

Lychee

Celery

Mango

Cucumbers

Melon

Eggplant

Oranges

Kale

Papaya

Lettuce

Passion Fruit

Okra

Pears

Onions

Plums

Spinach

Pomegranate

Tomatoes

Turnip Greens

Watercress

Zucchini

Healthy Fats

Your body requires an ample amount of unsaturated fats rich in omega-3. They contribute to maintaining skin hydration and radiance, supporting optimal cellular function, aiding in digestion, and potentially reducing inflammatory responses. These fats are essential for maintaining a lean physique.

Dietary recommendation: It is advised that 15 percent of your daily caloric intake consists of nutritious fats derived from sources such as nuts, seeds, healthy oils, and fish.

Almonds

Avocado oil

Cashews

Flax seed

Hazelnut oil

Olive oil

Pecans

Pumpkinseed oil

Safflower oil

Sunflower seeds

Walnuts

Coconut oil

The Rise And Notion Of Dietary Cleanliness

The concept of clean eating entails the belief that consuming primarily unprocessed, whole foods and avoiding refined sugar and other processed foods can greatly enhance one's overall health and well-being. In essence, it pertains to your ability to possess the steadfastness to cease indulging in nutritionally deficient substances."

Given that it is an efficacious method for enhancing one's overall quality of life, it is unsurprising to observe that fitness experts, nutrition professionals, and conscientious individuals have long embraced this advantageous dietary approach. It is important to acknowledge at this point that the concept of "clean eating" should not be regarded merely as a diet, but rather as a lifestyle that has been followed for centuries, predating the actual term.

In contemporary times, it has become increasingly commonplace to observe the endorsement and advocacy of this distinctive way of living by renowned personalities in the entertainment industry, such as Kate Perry, who is widely recognized as a prominent Hollywood figure. The concept of adhering to a wholesome dietary approach has consistently been associated with Ella Mills, Natasha Corrett, and the Hemsley sisters, despite their steadfast refutations of ever employing the specific terminology.

There are multiple iterations of this phenomenon that may necessitate the avoidance of dairy, gluten, grains, and even advocate for the consumption of uncooked food.

The Fundamental Tenets of Nutritious Consumption

Initially, it may seem that adhering to such a way of life is arduous, but upon deeper examination, one will realize that embracing its fundamental tenets is actually uncomplicated and direct. Several tenets associated with adhering to a clean eating lifestyle comprise the subsequent aspects:

• It is recommended to consume breakfast within an hour of awakening each morning on a daily basis.

• In order to regulate blood glucose levels and curb appetite, it is advisable to consume frequent, small meals approximately five times per day.

• Ensure that the foods you consume are unprocessed, maintaining their integrity throughout handling, packaging, and storage, and obtained directly from the farm. To provide an example, it is necessary for fruits, legumes, vegetables, and grains to remain unprocessed, whereas nuts and seeds should not have any added salt. Additionally, it is important for chickens to be raised in free-range conditions and for beef to be derived from grass-fed sources.

• It is recommended that you consume a minimum of 2 liters of water on a daily basis. or • It is advisable to ensure a daily water intake of at least 2 liters.

• Please ensure that your meals contain appropriate portions of lean protein, healthy fats, and complex carbohydrates.

• Avoid consuming processed or refined foods such as confections, sugary items, products made with white flour, white rice, etc.

• Avoid consuming foods that have low nutritional value and are high in calories, essentially referring to various forms of unhealthy processed foods.

• It is strongly advised to abstain from consuming beverages such as drinks, sodas, and juices that contain excessive calories but lack nutritional benefits for the body. Imagine a situation in which an individual becomes entangled in the detrimental practice of consuming a minimum of one bottle of soda each day, persisting over an extended period of time. Now, engage in profound contemplation regarding the potential harm that substances such as preservatives and refined sugars may be imposing upon his/her well-being.

• Utilize the opportunity provided by fresh fruits and vegetables to obtain dietary fiber, essential vitamins, vital nutrients, and beneficial enzymes for the enhancement of your body's well-being.

• Ensure proper portion control for each meal • Skillfully manage the serving sizes for all meals • Maintain appropriate portion sizes for every meal • Ensure that each meal is served with appropriate portion sizes • Supervise the portioning of every meal in a diligent manner.

• Refrain from excessive smoking and alcohol consumption.

• Endeavor to prepare your meals to the greatest extent feasible.

• Engage in regular physical activity that will contribute to maintaining your fitness and overall well-being

• Avoid elevating food to the level of worship • Refrain from idolizing food • Do not adulate or deify food • Exercise moderation and avoid excessive reverence towards food • Maintain a balanced and measured attitude towards food

• All activities must be carried out in moderation. • One should engage in everything in moderation. • It is important to exercise moderation in all endeavors. • All actions must be conducted with a sense of moderation. • Practicing moderation in all aspects is highly advised.

• Strive to find contentment in life without fixating on it excessively, while embracing moments of joy and pleasure.

Key Benefits of Embracing a Clean Eating Lifestyle

The essential inquiries that an individual who prioritizes their health may wish to pose is what benefits they can derive from consuming pure and wholesome sustenance. No matter what your intentions or motives may be regarding your desire to embrace clean eating, you will discover it to be an essential and fundamental component of a well-rounded lifestyle that will enhance your quality of life. The reasons behind the inclination to embrace a clean diet may stem from an aspiration to shed pounds, adopt a wholesome way of living, or maintain physical fitness as one progresses in age.

By adhering to a diet that primarily consists of nutritious, minimally processed foods such as fruits, nuts, seeds, fish, and lean meat, among other options, you will supply your body with the necessary nutrients required for optimal cellular functioning and the potential prevention of chronic illnesses. Furthermore, the removal of unhealthy foods from your diet yields substantial advantages, as the substances present in detrimental and processed foods have the potential to heighten your susceptibility to various ailments.

The notable benefits of consuming wholesome foods encompass the subsequent:

To enhance your energy levels" "To heighten your energy reserves" "To bolster your physical stamina" "To elevate your overall vitality" "To augment your levels of vigor" "To amplify your energy quotient

Consuming nourishing meals not only enhances your vitality and efficiency but aids in properly nurturing your physique. Several essential nutrients, such as B-complex vitamins and iron, provide the necessary fuel for cells to function optimally. Further advantages of consuming a nutritious diet include its role in the facilitation of blood sugar regulation, thereby mitigating the occurrence of surges in glucose levels that may precipitate fatigue. Consuming refined carbohydrates such as confectioneries frequently leads to the development of such health conditions.

Quick Tip 1

A highly effective approach for boosting your energy levels is to incorporate breakfasts that contain whole grains abundant in dietary fibers, thereby providing you with ample energy to sustain yourself until lunchtime.

Quick Tip 2

Food that has undergone denaturation or processing often lacks dietary fiber, which assists in the regulation of gastrointestinal issues like bloating and constipation. Therefore, it is advisable to consume a nutritious diet comprising of high-fiber foods in order to regulate bowel movements and prevent the occurrence of constipation.

It serves to alleviate the potential hazards associated with cardiovascular illnesses

By choosing to adhere to a lifestyle that centers on consuming a nutritious and uncontaminated diet, you are, to some extent, diminishing the likelihood of experiencing cardiovascular disease. As an instance, the substantial quantities of vitamin C found in a variety of fruits and vegetables play a pivotal role in fortifying blood vessels. Consequently, the consumption of these natural sources aids in reducing the risk of developing coronary heart disease and provides protection against conditions such as hypertension and cerebrovascular accidents.

It is of utmost importance to consider the fact that the incorporation of specific beneficial fats derived from plants, such as olive oil, coconut oil, and various nuts, has the propensity to diminish elevated levels of harmful cholesterol, thereby effectively mitigating the risk of cardiovascular disease. In contrast, a diet that is not conducive to overall well-being and is high in saturated fat is known to elevate blood cholesterol levels, thereby jeopardizing the health of your cardiovascular system.

Combats Cancer

Adhering to a nourishing diet provides significant support in combating the proliferation of cancer. It should not be unexpected to you that numerous studies have demonstrated that the consumption of processed foods high in saturated fat, plant-based imitations of meat, and fried foods can elevate the likelihood of developing cancer.

On the other hand, a healthful diet comprising an ample quantity of fruits and vegetables not only improves the assimilation of phytonutrients and antioxidants, but also plays a vital role in combatting cancer development.

Benefits Of Clean Eating

Clean eating is not a passing trend in dietary practices; rather, it constitutes a sustainable way of life that can offer numerous remarkable advantages to one's health, exemplified by the subsequent enumeration:

Boosts energy levels

Adhering to a wholesome and nourishing diet enhances your vitality and promotes heightened productivity. Vital nutrients such as iron and B-complex vitamins facilitate cellular access to sufficient energy, thereby enabling proper functionality of cells.

Clean eating additionally contributes to the regulation of blood sugar levels, thus diminishing the likelihood of experiencing sudden increases in blood sugar, commonly induced by the consumption of processed carbohydrates such as refined grains and sugary foods. To enhance your energy levels, commence your day with a nutrient-rich breakfast consisting of three indispensable elements: protein, nourishing fats, and whole grains that are brimming with fiber.

Enhances mood

A diet that is abundant in B-vitamins has been acknowledged for its ability to enhance the synthesis of serotonin and dopamine, which are neurotransmitters associated with positive emotions. Additionally, omega-3 fatty acids have been implicated in ameliorating depressive symptoms and preventing fluctuations in mood. In a research conducted in New Zealand, it was observed that increased intake of fruits and vegetables yielded a state of serenity and enhanced levels of overall happiness and wellbeing. Not only are these favorable effects observable on the days when individuals consume a higher proportion of real foods, but they also persist throughout the subsequent day.

Mitigates the likelihood of developing a range of illnesses.

Processed foods typically contain excessive amounts of fat, sugar, or sodium, leading to the introduction of superfluous additives and calories. These components have been closely linked to the development of chronic ailments such as diabetes, cardiovascular disorders, and specific types of cancer. The consumption of fruits and vegetables provides protection against hypertension and cerebrovascular accidents, whereas the consumption of healthful fats present in olive oil, avocados, and nuts mitigates the levels of detrimental cholesterol.

Aids in the stimulation of metabolism and facilitation of detoxification.

Adhering to a wholesome dietary regimen is the most effective approach to losing surplus weight without subjecting oneself to deprivation or adopting a rigid meal plan. Wholesome, unprocessed foods inherently possess reduced levels of salt, sugar, and fat, while remaining free from additives and synthetic constituents that may pose health risks. By adhering to a nutritious and balanced dietary regimen, it is possible to achieve a weight loss of up to 20 pounds within a matter of weeks, while also sustaining a desirable body weight for an extended period. Furthermore, the inherent constituents found in wholesome food items aid in the detoxification of your body, eliminating detrimental toxins and chemicals that may have accumulated within your system.

Improves brain function

The optimal functioning of the brain necessitates a well-calibrated blend of nutritive elements, including beneficial lipids, select carbohydrates, and vital nourishment. This ensures enhanced performance in various domains such as employment, academics, and day-to-day engagements. Based on a recent study conducted by the National Institute, it has been found that enhancing one's consumption of unadulterated, genuine food items like fruits, vegetables, fish, whole grains, avocado, beans, nuts, and seeds can diminish the likelihood of developing cerebral infarctions. These infarctions are characterized by minute zones of necrotic brain tissue and have been linked to cognitive impairments.

Combats cancer growth

Adhering to a wholesome dietary regimen aids in the restraint of cancer development, while consuming a diet predominantly consisting of processed edibles (especially fried foods, processed meat, packaged meals, and saturated fat) augments your susceptibility to cancer. Fruits and vegetables possess significant quantities of antioxidants and phytonutrients renowned for their capacity to combat cancer. Tomatoes and cruciferous vegetables, such as kale and broccoli, possess notable advantages.

Strengthens immune system

Nutrient-rich foods facilitate the enhancement of the body's immune system, bolstering its capacity to naturally combat illnesses and expedite recovery. A clean diet additionally enhances gut health, facilitating optimal nutrient assimilation while mitigating the likelihood of detrimental toxins infiltrating the bloodstream. The digestive system harbors an extensive array of over 500 distinct bacterial species, which serve the essential function of facilitating food digestion and maintaining the overall well-being of the intestinal tract. Probiotics, which are classified as beneficial microorganisms, are thought to contribute to immune system maintenance through the regulation of immune responses. In order to maintain optimal functioning of your immune system, it is advisable to ensure proper hydration and incorporate ample amounts of fermented foods, yogurt, as well as a diverse array of vibrant vegetables and fruits into your diet.

Yields a heightened sense of satisfaction

Consuming a nutritionally balanced diet that includes nourishing fats, whole-grain carbohydrates, and protein will supply your body with ample energy to sustain you for extended periods, affording your hunger signals a lengthier respite. These food items provide a heightened feeling of satiety and assist in preventing excessive consumption, thereby reducing the likelihood of experiencing bloating and gastrointestinal discomfort.

Promotes cell growth

A wholesome dietary regimen that incorporates compounds such as antioxidants, vitamins, minerals, and omega-3 fatty acids fosters optimal cellular development, thereby enhancing the vitality and resilience of your hair, nails, and skin. Proteins constitute the structural components of both nails and hair; therefore, it is important to incorporate beans, nuts, eggs, poultry, and fish into your dietary intake. Consuming a diverse selection of vegetables and fruits also enhances the presence of biotin and vitamins C and E in the body. These nutrients are vital for promoting strong nails, long hair, and maintaining a healthy and radiant complexion.

Enhances athletic performance

A diet comprising authentic, unprocessed foods will facilitate muscular development, enhance endurance, and nourish your cognitive functions, enabling sustained focus and heightened attentiveness. Tailoring your dietary choices to align with the specific sports you participate in, you have the option to incorporate food sources rich in protein, such as lean meats, fish, poultry, cheese, and eggs, into your nutrition regimen.

Promotes better dental health

By excluding sweetened beverages and sugary foods from your dietary intake, you can mitigate the likelihood of experiencing oral conditions such as gingivitis and dental caries, while simultaneously promoting a favorable oral environment. If one frequently experiences an insatiable desire for sweet-tasting items, it is advisable to opt for the naturally occurring sugars present in fruits. You have the option to combine them with Greek yogurt in order to satiate your desires. Yogurt also contains calcium, a mineral recognized for its ability to fortify dental structures.

Improves sleep

Nutrient-rich foods comprise essential vitamins and minerals that aid in regulating hormonal activity during the day and facilitate restful sleep during night hours. Nutritious dietary choices additionally elicit a soothing effect on the central nervous system and stimulate the release of sleep-promoting hormones, thereby facilitating improved quality and depth of sleep during nighttime. Foods that possess elevated levels of tryptophan, such as low-fat or skim milk and almonds, afford both melatonin and protein, thereby facilitating a rapid induction of sleep.

The quest for unadulterated, organic sustenance has become increasingly arduous in contemporary times, as the market is predominantly saturated with processed and packaged food products.

But should you exert additional effort to exclusively select authentic products, you shall not only reap these remarkable health advantages, but also an array of additional benefits!

Meal Planning And Recipes

Embarking on a clean eating journey might pose some initial difficulties. However, this chapter provides a comprehensive meal plan accompanied by a shopping list, thereby simplifying the process. The duration of the plan is set for a period of seven days. This will facilitate a smoother transition for you to manage.

Week One

"On Monday:

In the morning meal, we suggest preparing a Summer Omelet by gently frying two finely chopped green onions, a quarter cup of finely chopped fennel, one cup of finely chopped Swiss chard, and a tablespoon of... Using 2 teaspoons, combine a quantity of chopped dill, a sprinkle of salt, and a sprinkle of pepper. comprised of premium-quality virgin olive oil. Incorporate four eggs into the mixture and proceed to whisk them together with one teaspoon. of water. Prepare the egg and execute a single flip. Consume only fifty percent of the omelets and retain the remainder. Consume it alongside a portion of ½ cup of cherries and a single slice of whole wheat bread.

"○ Refreshments: A single peach and a half ounce of walnuts

Menu Option: Halloumi Salad is prepared by combining grilled Halloumi, cut into cubes measuring 2 ounces, with ½ cup of chickpeas, ¼ cup of chopped cucumbers, sliced tomatoes, and 1 tablespoon of dressing. consisting of a hint of mint, a touch of parsley, and a sprinkle of dill. Incorporate one cup of arugula along with two teaspoons. consisting of additional virgin olive oil combined with a hint of lemon juice. Incorporate a small amount of salt and a small amount of pepper. Accompany it with a three-ounce portion of tuna.

○ Snack portion: 2 tablespoons. Comprised of a portion of Edamame hummus accompanied by half of a cucumber, expertly prepared into stick-like shapes.

○ Dinner: Enjoy a single portion of curried apricot pan-roasted chicken dish

- consume half and reserve the remainder

"● On Tuesday:

○ Morning Meal: Strawberry Mint Smoothie: Combine 1 cup of kefir, 1 cup of strawberries, 2 tablespoons of mint, half a cup of ice, and 1 teaspoon. of honey, 1 tsp. consisting of vanilla extract and a quantity of 2 tablespoons of hemp seeds. Consume just half of the serving and proceed to deposit the remainder into a Popsicle mold for preservation - Pair it alongside a singular slice of bread that has been spread with a measured quantity of 2 tablespoons of peanut butter.

"○ Mid-afternoon refreshment: Consume a portion of Edamame hummus measuring 2 tablespoons alongside half of a cucumber, cut into stick-shaped pieces.

○ Midday Meal: Savor the remaining Summer Omelets by pairing them with ½ cup of cooked farro and 1 succulent peach.

○ Refreshment: One ounce of walnuts accompanied by half a cup of cherries.

Dinner will consist of Open Faced Veggie Melts topped with Smoked Mozzarella.

"● The third day of the week, namely Wednesday:

○ Morning Meal Option: Cherry Farro Parfait: Utilizing a parfait-style vessel, carefully layer ⅔ cup of cooked farro, 1 tablespoon of finely chopped walnuts, ½ cup of sliced pitted cherries, ½ cup of kefir, and 1 teaspoon. Two teaspoons of hemp seeds. Consisting of a quantity of honey, alongside a hint of cinnamon, and complemented by a touch of nutmeg.

- Snack: Consume 2 tablespoons of edamame hummus alongside half a cup of fennel slices.

Lunch: A single portion of leftover Curried Apricot Pan Roasted Chicken.

○ Snack: Two teaspoons. Spread a generous layer of peanut butter onto half of a bread slice. After toasting, lightly dust it with a blend of cinnamon and nutmeg.

○ Dinner: Grilled Barramundi with Herb Sauce: Begin by preparing the asparagus bunch, ensuring to trim it and subsequently coating it with a generous 2 tsp. composed of extra virgin olive oil, a pinch of salt, and a pinch of pepper. Cook it over an open flame using the zest derived from a singular lemon. Consume four of the asparagus stalks and reserve the remaining portion. Consume it alongside a serving of 1 cup of quinoa.

Thursday: ● Upon the arrival of the fourth day of the week,...

○ Morning Meal: Green Egg Benedict: Incorporate 4 remaining asparagus spears, along with 3 slices of avocado, crowned with an egg cooked over easy using a half teaspoon of oil. comprised of extra virgin olive oil. Apply a quarter portion of the remaining herb sauce as a drizzle.

○ Afternoon Refreshment: Layer half a cup of kefir with half a cup of sliced strawberries. Drizzle on 1 tsp. of honey.

○ Midday Meal: Prepare a nourishing Strawberry Kale Salad by combining a generous portion of 2 cups of baby kale with a delicate ½ cup of sliced strawberries and cooked farro. Enhance the flavors by adding 1 ounce of grilled and diced Halloumi cheese. Incorporate 1 tablespoon of pistachios. Whisk 2 tsp. one teaspoon of extra virgin olive oil half a teaspoon of balsamic vinegar consisting of a measure of honey, a hint of salt, and a touch of pepper. Drizzle on the salad. Consume it alongside a single portion of whole wheat bread.

o Snack: Two teaspoons. a dollop of peanut butter on the surface of a half portion of a sliced peach.

o Dinner: One portion of leftover curried apricot pan roasted chicken.

"● On Friday:

o Breakfast: Avocado Puree with Hemp Seeds: Spread ¼ portion of mashed avocado onto a single slice of bread, and delicately sprinkle it with 2 teaspoons of hemp seeds. Consisting of a quarter teaspoon of hemp seeds. consisting of grated lemon peel along with a pinch of salt and a pinch of pepper. Consume it in conjunction with a serving of cherries.

- Snack: one teaspoon. - Snack portion: one teaspoon. - A teaspoon serving size of snack. A serving of leftover edamame hummus accompanied by four asparagus spears.

Lunch: Prepare a Halloumi Salad by combining 2 ounces of grilled Halloumi, cubed, with ½ cup of chickpeas, ¼ cup of cucumbers and sliced tomatoes, as well as 1 tablespoon of finely chopped mint, dill, and parsley. Incorporate 1 cup of arugula in conjunction with 21 teaspoons. Comprising a measured quantity of extra virgin olive oil, a squeeze of fresh lemon juice, a sprinkle of salt, and a sprinkle of pepper. Accompany it with a three-ounce portion of tuna. Eat the Popsicle.

o Midday Nourishment: A modest portion of fennel, about a half cup, delicately coated with a quarter portion of remaining herbal sauce.

o Evening Meal: Mediterranean Quinoa

On Saturday:

o Breakfast: A nourishing Strawberry Farro Bowl consisting of 1 cup of cooked Farro paired with ½ cup of kefir, ½ cup of sliced strawberries, and a garnish of 2 tablespoons of chopped almonds. Finish by delicately drizzling the dish with 1 teaspoon. of honey and mint. Sprinkle it with a combination of cinnamon and nutmeg.

o Light refreshment: One half portion of bread accompanied by two teaspoons.

consisting of a serving of edamame hummus accompanied by a quarter cup of sliced cherry tomatoes

Lunch will consist of leftover Mediterranean Quinoa.

○ Midday nourishment: Consume a serving of 1 ounce of walnuts in conjunction with a singular orange.

The evening meal consists of a deliciously prepared steak accompanied by Romaine hearts and a tangy date sauce.

• Sunday:

○ Breakfast: Nutritious Green Eggs: Gently cook 2 cups of kale in 2 tsp. Incorporate a tablespoon of extra virgin olive oil, along with a clove of minced garlic, totaling two teaspoons. Consisting of finely diced dill and parsley, a finely chopped green onion, a small pinch of salt, and a subtle sprinkle of pepper. Relocate it onto a plate and subsequently proceed to whisk two eggs within the very same cooking utensil. Consume it accompanied by half of a peach.

○ Afternoon Refreshment: Enjoy a serving of kefir accompanied by one ounce of toasted almonds. Gently incorporate a small amount of nutmeg and cinnamon on top. Consume it alongside 1/4 cup of cherries

○ Lunch: Sea and Pea Salad: Mix together 2 ounces of tuna, ½ cup of chickpeas, and 1 finely diced green onion. Equal amounts of diced cucumber, alongside an equivalent quantity of sliced tomatoes. Add in 2 tsp. one teaspoon of extra virgin olive oil comprising of one tablespoon of lemon juice of dill and parsley. Consume it in conjunction with a single piece of bread.

o Snack: One-half portion of bread containing two teaspoons. consisting of a portion of edamame hummus and one-fourth of the herb sauce.

o Dinner: Remaining portion of Mediterranean Quinoa

Health Benefits

On a daily basis, the typical American individual ingests approximately 2700 calories and 126 grams of sugar. The prescribed daily allowances amount to 2000 and 25, correspondingly. Naturally, the daily caloric requirements may vary among individuals, nonetheless, the prevailing obesity epidemic (with over 60% of Americans classified as overweight) does exemplify the necessity for calorie limitation quite effectively.

However, it is not solely limited to caloric restriction. Increased consumption of sugar, particularly that derived from processed and refined sources, is strongly correlated with an elevation in body weight. The rise of fast food establishments and the proliferation of highly processed food containing excessive amounts of fats and sugars are predominantly responsible for the widespread obesity crisis, leaving little room for skepticism. A diet consisting of unprocessed, nutrient-rich foods effectively circumvents the challenges that afflict a significant majority of American individuals and a substantial portion of the global population.

I concur wholeheartedly with the USDA's fundamental suggestion regarding the composition of an ordinary dinner. An optimal allocation of space on your plate would dictate that fifty percent should be dedicated to vegetables or fruit. The remaining portions ought to consist of protein and grain.

Please take into account the following arrangement: a plate consisting of one cup of cooked red beans, one cup of brown rice, and two cups of the Bird's Eye Normandy blend appears as described. Following are the nutritional values: a total of 446 calories, consisting of 40 grams of protein, meeting 4% of your recommended daily sodium intake, accompanied by 8 grams of sugar and 2 grams of fat.

If one opts to abstain from using whole ingredients and instead source each element of the meal from manufacturers (such as Blue Runner beans, Uncle Ben's rice, Del Monte mixed vegetables), here is the resulting outcome. The food item contains 630 calories, 14 grams of sugar, a substantial 71% of the recommended sodium intake, 5 grams of fat, and merely 31 grams of protein. Furthermore, one must also consider the implications regarding the presence of preservatives and the associated concerns with regard to the preparation process.

The entire process of food preparation comprises reduced calorie content, approximately half the amount of sugar, less than half the quantity of fat, and less than one twentieth of the sodium content. It is evident that there exists a discernible distinction.

This is a highly straightforward illustration, yet it effectively exemplifies the point. Devoting greater focus towards the quality and composition of food products during the purchasing process holds substantial potential to accrue considerable advantages for you. Moreover, if you eliminate pre-prepared food altogether and solely rely on whole ingredients, this becomes even more significant. Conduct thorough investigations on the companies from which you make purchases, acquire knowledge about their methodologies and operational structures, and gain a comprehensive understanding of the origins of your food. It is of utmost importance.

Engage In Smart Meal Preparation And Consider Healthier Eating Options

One of the initial steps required to initiate your clean eating regimen entails thoroughly inspecting and modifying the contents of your pantry to align with your newfound dietary preferences. During the process of organizing your pantry, you may have discerned the presence of a notable quantity of 'comestibles' that are not in a state of cleanliness. To establish a pantry conducive to maintaining a wholesome diet, it is imperative to eliminate all items considered "unwholesome" to prevent relapse into previous dietary patterns.

If it is not financially viable to discard all of these food items and begin anew, an alternative approach would be to gradually substitute these unhealthy foods with those comprised of clean ingredients, one at a time. Through this practice, you mitigate food wastage while gradually transforming your pantry.

Crucial Staples for Nourishing a Healthy Eating Cupboard

Now that you have made the necessary preparations to maintain a more nutritious pantry, it is imperative to acquire knowledge regarding the strategies employed by those who adhere to clean eating principles, particularly when it comes to meal planning, grocery shopping, and pantry management. Prior to delving into the intricacies of meal planning, it is imperative that we initially ascertain the customary ingredients employed in clean eating recipes.

To begin with, it is important to ensure that your pantry is stocked with whole wheat pastry flour. This particular type of flour serves as the most optimal alternative to white flour. Regardless of your interest in baking, it becomes evident that recipes frequently call for white flour in order to prepare meals for both lunch and dinner, or to create delectable desserts. In addition to its application in baking, white flour functions as a means of thickening sauces or as a coating for deep-frying purposes.

The subsequent item of sustenance is beans. This food is filled with a plethora of essential vitamins and minerals. Furthermore, they can be incorporated into a multitude of culinary preparations. Beans are frequently found in a variety of culinary preparations, including salads, soups, and vegetable side dishes. You are afforded the choice between purchasing fresh or canned beans. Ensure that you verify the contents listed on the ingredient list for any items that are forbidden. Several prevalent varieties of beans include chickpeas, kidney beans, black beans, adzuki beans, pinto beans, and navy beans.

Other significant food items include grains, dairy substitutes, and nuts. Prior to adopting a clean eating regimen, my knowledge of grains was limited to rice, oats, and wheat. Due to adhering to a clean eating regimen, I have had the pleasure of exploring and relishing in an array of diverse grain selections, including but not limited to quinoa, brown rice, barley, millet, amaranth, faro, buckwheat, and oats.

In regards to dairy substitutes, I employ almond milk, rice milk, hemp milk, and hazelnut milk (all devoid of sweeteners) to substitute conventional dairy items. Nuts prove to be quite useful, particularly when it comes to snacking. This particular category of food item is abundant in essential nutrients and enhances the taste of any culinary creation. Almonds, hazelnuts, walnuts, and pecans are among the frequently utilized nuts that would be indispensable additions to your pantry.

If one possesses a fondness for confections akin to my own, it would be wise to perpetually maintain a stock of these alternative sweetening agents within the confines of one's pantry, so as to ensure a ready supply for the creation of delectable desserts and other indulgent delicacies. Dear, Sucanat, maple syrup, brown rice syrup, and liquid stevia are frequently utilized as substitutes for sugar in various cooking and baking applications.

In order to assist you in devising your shopping list, presented herein are the essential 50 food items that are imperative for well-stocked clean eating pantries.

Apples

Asparagus

Artichokes

Apricots

Avocados

Beans and legumes

Bananas

Beets

Blueberries

Broccoli

Brussels sprouts

Cauliflower

Cabbage

Carrots

Cherries

Cantaloupe

Cranberries

Chia Seeds

Flax

Fish

Eggs

Dark Chocolate

Greek yogurt

Grapes

Garlic

Green Tea

Kale

Kiwi

Oats

Nuts

Lemons

Mushrooms

Mangoes

Peaches

Papaya

Pineapple

Oranges

Olive Oil

Pumpkin

Quinoa

Pomegranates

Brown Rice

Wild Salmon

Spinach

Swiss chard

Sweet potatoes

Tomatoes

Wheat germ

Watermelon

Winter Squash

How to Shop

Now that you have acquired knowledge regarding which foods to seek out, it is appropriate to conceive a strategy for conducting a streamlined shopping experience. At this point in time, it is expected that you possess knowledge concerning the types of food that meet the criteria for being considered clean, as well as the factors to consider when examining food labels. In order to alleviate anxiety and conserve valuable time during your initial grocery expedition as a practitioner of clean eating, it is imperative to keep in mind five essential suggestions.

Firstly, fresh food items can invariably be located in the periphery of supermarkets. If you are in pursuit of fresh culinary provisions, simply proceed by pulling your carriage and adhering to the walls. In that location, one can discover a range of offerings such as newly sourced meat and produce, along with an array of dairy products, not to mention the inclusion of a deli and bakery section. If you are able to refrain from visiting the delicatessen and bakery, you will fare satisfactorily.

Secondly, it is important to observe and make note of the aisles in the vicinity. Given your commitment to maintaining a clean eating regimen, it would be prudent to refrain from perusing the aisles. Acquaint yourself with the aisles housing canned vegetables and broths, grain products, as well as organic foods, and confine your shopping exclusively to those aisles until you become adept at purchasing natural and unprocessed food items. In addition to the supermarket, it would be advantageous to explore alternative options such as patronizing your neighborhood butcher and an establishment specializing in organic food products, in order to expand your shopping prospects.

Thirdly, it is advisable to refrain from engaging in shopping activities while experiencing hunger. Indeed, this principle is also applicable to individuals who adhere to clean eating practices. Impulsive shopping frequently occurs when individuals make food purchases while experiencing hunger. This frequently leads to the purchase of unhealthy snack items or food items that do not align with one's desired dietary choices. Prior to your departure, I would recommend creating a detailed shopping list and adhering to it. Not only will you experience an improvement in your overall well-being, but you will also realize fiscal benefits.

Fourthly, if you are afforded the opportunity, do not hesitate to venture into alternative sections. In such circumstances, one can engage in the exercise of scrutinizing product labels, thereby identifying alternate nourishing options that can be incorporated into their meals.

Fifthly, endeavor to make purchases in larger quantities whenever possible. Purchasing food items in large quantities results in cost and time savings. Another worthwhile suggestion is to explore the extensive selection of ingredients available in the bulk section of the supermarket. This section offers a wide range of items that you may not have had the opportunity to experiment with previously.

Utilize The Principles Of Clean Eating To Benefit Your Health

The clean eating lifestyle can be adopted by individuals of all backgrounds, allowing them to gradually modify their dietary choices to incorporate healthier food options. In this instance, a high level of dedication is of utmost importance for an individual such as yourself, to ensure unwavering commitment to your endeavors. This will furnish you with the necessary impetus to remain steadfast and accomplish your objectives, whether it pertains to weight reduction or pursuing other health-related goals.

You can effectively incorporate a clean eating regimen into your lifestyle. Outlined below are several recommended actions that can aid in alleviating bloating, reducing weight, and progressing towards a more slender and vigorous version of yourself. Additionally, a compilation of unfavorable practices to steer clear of is also provided.

Avoiding Common Mistakes

When considering any subsequent alteration in one's lifestyle, it is imperative to allow for the occurrence of errors or missteps. Simply gather yourself, remove any remnants of setback, and make another attempt. Additionally, it would be advantageous to possess a compendium of typical errors often made by individuals who are inexperienced in adhering to a clean eating regimen.

By gaining insight into the challenges encountered by others, it may facilitate your ability to circumvent these mistakes.

Failing to moderate your eating speed

The brain typically requires approximately 20 minutes to perceive the sensation of satiety as the stomach gradually becomes filled with food.

Should you engage in rapid consumption of food, it is plausible to ingest a substantial quantity of calories unknowingly, resulting in a persistent sense of dissatisfaction despite the copious amount of sustenance already consumed.

By engaging in deliberate mastication and adopting a more measured pace when consuming each mouthful, individuals can effectively reduce their caloric intake by refraining from consuming unnecessary excess food, all the while alleviating the burden on their digestive system.

Enforcing overly stringent dietary restrictions.

If an excessive number of dietary restrictions are imposed, the long-term viability of the regimen may be compromised. Numerous individuals experience failure as a consequence of fixating on minutiae. If your priority is to modify your dietary habits, it is imperative that you afford yourself the opportunity to acclimate to and adapt new methodologies.

It would also be beneficial if you allocate even a marginal portion of your dietary consumption to accommodate the foods that you derive pleasure from eating. By doing this, you will find increased motivation to adhere to a clean eating regimen for an extended duration.

Inconsistency

Consistency plays a pivotal role in attaining the desired outcomes in any endeavor you undertake. While the notion of gradually adopting clean eating habits has been put forth, it is crucially important that as you advance, your primary emphasis should lie on incorporating a greater quantity of nutritious food into your diet.

Attempt to gradually overcome the tendency to consume a substantial breakfast, only to subsequently follow it with fast food meals throughout the entirety of the day.

Accumulating the cereals

The human body necessitates the inclusion of grains in one's diet, as they serve as crucial sources of carbohydrates, fiber, and even protein. It is imperative, however, to maintain moderation in consumption, as excessive intake of any substance is ill-advised. Particularly in the case of unprocessed grains, albeit their superiority over refined grains, excessive consumption may contribute to weight gain.

Engaging in late-day carbohydrate loading

It is customary for individuals who are new to dieting to adhere to their regimen during early hours, only to indulge in excessive eating later in the evening. The identical occurrence transpires when one embarks on a nutritious dietary regimen.

As one's determination weakens over the course of the day, there is a tendency to become vulnerable to consuming significant quantities of unhealthy carbohydrates, particularly ones derived from white flour and sugar, which the body subsequently converts into fat deposits.

Not reading labels

Despite the legal requirement for the inclusion of nutritional information on all packaged food items, this remains one of the most overlooked aspects worldwide. Within the realm of healthy eating, there is no space for careless presumptions. It is of utmost significance that you possess knowledge regarding the constituents of the edibles you are about to consume.

Not reading food labels is a grave error. Despite the labeling of certain products as healthy, low-fat, low-sodium, or similar claims, it is important to note that these items often contain chemical constituents that may deviate from the principles of clean eating. Additionally, it is worth noting that the product label provides essential details regarding the calorie content of the food item. This information holds significant importance, particularly for individuals who are diligently monitoring their caloric intake. Do not allow an occurrence that is quite literally within your immediate vicinity serve as the cause of your failure.

Concentrating on a singular category of wholesome sustenance at a given time.

When initiating a regimen of clean eating, endeavor to fully embrace the entire process rather than selectively incorporating certain aspects of it.

Rather than prioritizing the consumption of whole grains, fruits, and vegetables, it would be advisable to dedicate a portion of your time and energy towards the meticulous selection of nutritious and well-rounded meals. As previously stated, it is imperative that each meal comprises essential components such as protein, fats, carbohydrates, dietary fibers, fruits, and vegetables.

Failing to properly address and manage cravings and sensations of hunger.

When embracing a clean eating regimen, one will transition to consuming smaller, more frequent meals throughout the course of the day. This aids in alleviating hunger pangs induced by alternative dietary plans. However, it is important to acknowledge that there may be occasions when your body craves additional nourishment, and mishandling these impulses can result in significant weight increase.

In many instances, individuals who perceive themselves as hungry despite consuming a complete meal are, in fact, undergoing a state of dehydration. In the event of experiencing hunger pangs, it is advisable to consume a glass of water. If this does not rectify the situation, consider consuming a serving of fresh produce. Please refrain from hurriedly moving through the kitchen in pursuit of the bag of cookies.

Developing an Understanding of Caloric
Intake

In addition to exercising dietary caution,
it is advisable to commence the practice
of quantifying meal portions and caloric
intake. Keeping meticulous track of your
daily calorie intake represents an
efficacious approach to maintaining
adherence to one's clean eating regimen.
Please consider that, although
consuming higher quality food, it
remains imperative to restrict the
quantity of food you consume. In this
particular scenario, excessive
consumption of food remains a catalyst
for substantial increase in body weight.

Engaging in caloric calculations can be a straightforward endeavor. Currently, a multitude of applications are available for individuals to monitor their daily caloric intake and expenditure. For a traditional approach, consider carrying a pen and paper at all times to diligently note down your daily meals, even the most minimal, such as a small serving of almonds.

Maintaining accurate documentation is of paramount importance in this particular scenario. If the application is installed on your device, it will automatically transform the information you input about your food into estimated quantities of calories. If you opt to employ the traditional pen and paper method, you may manually perform the task by accessing an online conversion chart. To the greatest extent feasible, facilitate the tracking of calorie intake by opting for a digital solution. Ensure the app is installed on your mobile device or have a program downloaded onto your personal computer.

There are recommended guidelines available regarding the required daily calorie intake based on factors such as height, weight, gender, and level of physical activity. Additionally, there are online sources available that provide information on the recommended caloric intake or expenditure to achieve a specific weight goal.

Many individuals choose not to track their calorie intake due to the perceived time-consuming nature of the task. To overcome this challenge, it is recommended that you utilize contemporary advancements available to effortlessly manage calorie counting.

Guidelines to Initiate Your Journey

The primary aim of adhering to a clean eating regimen entails the adoption of a more healthful dietary intake, forsaking detrimental food choices for those that promote well-being. As you make improvements to your dietary habits, redirect your attention towards consuming a greater proportion of unprocessed, whole foods and fresh produce, rather than opting for their processed alternatives. Clean eating offers a multitude of advantages and embarking on this lifestyle shift is quite accessible.

Please articulate a rationale for your desire to commence consuming healthful, unprocessed foods.

The majority of individuals possess underlying motivations for their pursuits, and understanding the true rationale for embarking on a healthier eating regimen can serve as a formidable source of inspiration during moments of temptation to abandon one's goals.

To triumph in ventures unexplored, one must exert greater diligence and exertion. Having a wellspring of inspiration at your disposal would facilitate the achievement of every task. In this scenario, it is crucial that your fundamental motive for desiring to consume nutritious food is to enhance your overall well-being. Direct your attention towards the rationale behind the change, emphasizing how it will yield advantageous outcomes, thereby increasing your likelihood of success.

Determine the extent of dedication and commitment you are prepared to invest in order to achieve success.

Once you have determined the underlying motivations for desiring a clean diet, establish a level of dedication that you can consistently maintain. Please be aware that you are engaging in a process that entails a comprehensive transformation of your dietary patterns. Would you be able to engage in the task of preparing at least one meal per day for a week, as a means of initiating the process of home-cooking? Would you be able to allocate a minimum of 30 minutes per day for physical activity?

Do not overburden yourself in the initial stages. It bears resemblance to the process of goal setting, in which one must ascertain attainable levels of dedication that can be faithfully adhered to upon embarking on the path to improved dietary habits. Some individuals will achieve this goal immediately, while others may require additional time to reach it.

Evaluate your present dietary patterns, encompassing your daily intake.

If you have a comprehensive breakdown of your current dietary patterns, it will enable you to identify the specific elements that require modification.

Engage in this activity for a duration of approximately one to two weeks. Please record your daily food intake, whether it consists of an apple or a package of cookies. Please provide details regarding the specific times during the day when you consume meals. Take diligent notes to enhance your capacity to evaluate the magnitude of your dietary circumstances more effectively. This will aid you in identifying the aspects you should decrease or increase in consumption.

You have the option to download and install food journal applications onto your mobile device, or alternatively, employ a traditional method utilizing pen and paper, selecting whichever approach is most suitable to your preference and ease of use. Upon completing the preliminary documentation, conduct a thorough evaluation and compile three distinct catalogs: 1) food items to reduce consumption of, 2) food items to incorporate into your dietary regimen, and 3) food items worth contemplating the complete elimination of. The magnitude of these lists, whether they are extensive or limited in scope, will serve to mentally equip you for the forthcoming endeavor. This will effectively illustrate the extent to which a transformative adjustment in lifestyle is necessitated.

Establish your objectives and discern precise benchmarks.

Establish attainable objectives that are within your capabilities and can be accomplished incrementally. One may generate lists of objectives that are either short-term or long-term in nature, but it is advisable to commence with short-term objectives at this juncture. Furthermore, it is advisable to establish multiple intermediary objectives that serve as building blocks towards the ultimate long-term goal. This approach enables one to achieve significant milestones incrementally, alleviating the perception of an overwhelming task while sustaining high levels of motivation. Utilizing the lists you have prepared, engage in the selection and adjustment of various ingredients, incorporating or excluding them from your daily dietary regimen. In this situation, a gradual advancement would be preferable since it would not impose excessive pressure on you.

Start shopping smarter.

When you embark upon a visit to the market, exercise prudent consumer behavior. This entails the careful examination of labels and refraining from haste when locating ingredients. Evaluating the items you select for purchase will enhance your abilities as a discerning consumer of food. If feasible, establish an alternative pathway, specifically designed to guide you towards the section containing fresh food items, rather than towards the aisle dedicated to snacks. By following this approach, you can avoid placing yourself in situations of temptation.

Examine product labels, and if you encounter an abundance of ingredients that are difficult to articulate or spell, it is advised to remove said item. Do not be discouraged by the cost of organic products when considering your purchases. Indeed, although superior ingredients may have a higher cost, they will ultimately result in considerable savings in terms of medical expenses in the long run. Please exercise due diligence in considering your choices of food items. The process of selecting and procuring these ingredients holds utmost significance when pursuing a clean eating regimen. Devoid of adequate tools, no proficient artisan can successfully complete a task, and the same principle applies to you and your dietary needs.

Adopt the practice of meal prepping and focus on maintaining a wholesome diet.

When endeavoring to maintain a healthy eating regimen, it is imperative to allocate time to meticulously prepare your daily meals within the confines of your own residence. By allocating a few hours of your daily schedule, you can procure a receptacle adequately stocked with meals for the subsequent day. Regardless of your workplace setting, you will consistently have the pleasure of relishing a nourishing meal prepared at home, using ingredients that you possess complete knowledge of.

Initially, this will undeniably require a certain amount of time investment; however, once you become acquainted with the process, you may even endeavor to engage in meal prepping for prolonged periods, spanning several weeks. Envision the ability to effortlessly create a week's worth of culinary delights within a concise time frame. When it comes to culinary instructions, a plethora of them can be readily accessed on the internet, and certain websites even offer the convenience of generating a curated compilation of recipes tailored to your preferences. Additionally, there are smartphone applications available that offer the functionality to calculate preparation durations and calorie counts.

However, it is comprehensible that occasions may arise when it is necessary to engage in social activities and dine elsewhere. If it is feasible for you to transport a home-cooked meal, kindly feel free to avail yourself of this opportunity. However, if you are unable to do so, it would be advisable to carefully consider your choices when selecting what to order. The majority of restaurants nowadays offer great levels of accommodation. Alternatively, you have the option to request the staff to omit specific ingredients or have them served separately as per your preference. As previously mentioned, adhering to clean eating entails adopting a new way of life. However, it is important to note that embracing this approach need not entail excessively restricting one's daily activities.

Exploring The Relationship Between Metabolism And Clean Eating

In the introductory section, I provided a succinct overview of the issue surrounding the abundance of conflicting information within diverse dietary regimens aimed at weight loss.

I endeavored to underscore that the concept of the eating clean diet plan diverges from the conventional notion of a rigid focus solely on achieving a specific weight loss goal within a predetermined timeframe.

Now I would like to provide you with additional information regarding reasons why you can dismiss a significant portion of the discussion, which at times may resemble a competition focused on the trendiest or most popular diet at any given moment.

In the following chapter, I will provide you with a comprehensive set of impartial recommendations to enable you to make an informed selection of the most suitable clean eating dietary plan that aligns with your personal preferences and accommodates the dietary needs of your entire household.

The crucial aspect in selecting an appropriate dietary regimen is to acquire substantial knowledge on the intricacies of one's metabolic processes. After achieving proficiency in this skill, the process of identifying the most convenient methods for procuring and creating nutritious meals becomes rather straightforward.

It is pertinent to understand the physiological process wherein the human body converts caloric intake into energy, as well as the significance of carbohydrates and fats.

Let us commence by delving into the comprehension of the mechanisms through which your body metabolizes calories, subsequently transforming them into energy.

Essentially, the crux of the matter lies in energy. Whether it pertains to the activation of an incandescent bulb or the sustenance of one's physiological functions, an adequate supply of energy is imperative.

While an electric light bulb operates through the consumption of electricity, the human body functions through the utilization of bio-energy.

Our physical organisms are naturally attuned to efficiently transform various food sources into readily usable bio-energy. The phenomenon of transforming nourishment into vitality is frequently known as metabolism.

The process of glucose breakdown to produce Adenosine Triphosphate (ATP) is facilitated by our metabolism, thereafter utilized by an energy center inherent in every cell throughout our body.

Consequently, through the process of metabolism, the human body derives adenosine triphosphate (ATP) from ingested nutrients, serving as the crucial cellular fuel for energy production. Notably, the energy content of a given food item is assessed in terms of its calorie content.

In a broad sense, energy is derived from sources such as sugars, carbohydrates, or lipids. Nevertheless, it should be noted that these energy sources do not possess uniform levels of value.

We possess a collective understanding of sugars, carbohydrates, and fats. However, it is worthwhile to scrutinize it more closely.

In essence, pertaining to the physical constitution, several varieties of sugars can be identified. The three primary types present are glucose, fructose, and sucrose.

Glucose is the carbohydrate derivative that predominantly exists within the chemical composition of carbohydrates. Carbohydrates are often pleasing to the palate, although they encompass items composed of refined flour.

Glucose can be derived from a multitude of sources. It can originate from lipids, amino acids, or a wide range of other food sources.

Now we can proceed to examine the significance of calorie counting in upholding a state of optimal physical well-being. However, it is important to bear in mind that the sole focus on calorie counting does not encompass all aspects of developing a well-rounded dietary regimen.

Calorie counting is a valuable approach in order to monitor and gain insight into the typical upper limit of calories that should be consumed per meal.

The allocation of calories among various food groups and the distribution of total daily caloric intake across meals are wholly contingent upon individual requirements and lifestyle choices.

The crucial aspect lies in recognizing that the accumulation of surplus calories as fat is contingent upon comprehending the connection between overall caloric consumption and expenditure.

Therefore, should the overall daily caloric consumption surpass the body's total caloric expenditure, weight gain will transpire. When an insufficient quantity of calories is supplied to the body, it will undergo the process of metabolizing stored fat, resulting in weight reduction.

Nevertheless, when it comes to clean eating, the emphasis lies not primarily on weight reduction, but rather on ensuring that the body receives the precise caloric intake that aligns with one's lifestyle, all the while maintaining a nourishing blend of various food groups.

The optimal combination is determined exclusively by the quantity of calories expended during the course of your day.

If I expend a total of 2,250 calories daily but consume 2,540 calories, it follows that the surplus calories are deposited in my body as adipose tissue. Alternatively, in the event that my daily caloric expenditure is 2,625 calories while my daily caloric intake amounts to 2,800 calories, it is highly probable that I will obtain the surplus calories through the utilization of fat stores.

The human body never expends fuel (ATP) in vain; rather, it conserves it by converting it into adipose tissue. In cases of ATP deficiency, the body proceeds to acquire it by metabolizing either fat or muscle tissue.

How to Achieve Dietary Balance While Tracking Caloric Intake

At this point, you possess a comprehensive comprehension of metabolism and the significance of determining the average caloric expenditure throughout a typical day.

The clean eating philosophy revolves around the objective of meticulously crafting meals that provide the optimal amount of calories derived from nutritious and wholesome foods.

Nevertheless, rest assured that in the event that you are unfamiliar with the method of determining this numerical value independently, there is no cause for concern.

It's really simple.

It is imperative to acquire knowledge regarding two crucial concepts, namely, basal metabolic rate (BMR) and active metabolic rate (AMR).

Basal Metabolic Rate (BMR) refers to the pace at which calories are expended during periods of minimal activity, involving a state of rest and relaxation with a lack of significant physical exertion. Even during periods of physical inactivity, the body continues to expend energy through calorie consumption.

The Accelerated Metabolic Rate (AMR) corresponds to the increased caloric expenditure associated with physical activity as compared to a sedentary state.

It is highly probable that your AMR number will be utilized for the purpose of establishing a daily dietary regimen.

Please be aware that there could potentially be significant variations in your Adjustable Rate Mortgage on a daily basis.

An individual employed in an office setting, engaging in sedentary activities from the hours of 9 a.m. to 5 p.m., and exhibiting only moderate physical activity throughout the course of the work week, will demonstrate varying Active Metabolic Rates (AMRs) between weekdays and weekends, as a result of their gym attendance and increased physical exertion during the latter.

Are you beginning to comprehend the notion that clean eating does not adhere to a universal diet plan?

The concept of clean eating revolves around discovering the nourishing foods that align with your personal preferences, while ensuring a balanced combination of food groups, in appropriate amounts, consumed at the optimal moments.

You possess complete authority over the selection and quantity of food deciding to consume.

To ascertain your AMR and BMR, kindly record the relevant numerical values and proceed to input said values into the following equations.

"To determine the AMR for women, employing the subsequent formula:

The Basal Metabolic Rate (BMR) can be calculated using the following formula: 655 plus 4.35 multiplied by the weight in pounds, plus 4.7 multiplied by the height in inches, minus 4.7 multiplied by the age in years.

To ascertain the AMR for men, utilize the ensuing equation:

The Basal Metabolic Rate (BMR) can be calculated as follows: 66 multiplied by the weight in pounds, added to 12.7 multiplied by the height in inches, and then subtracting 6.8 multiplied by the age.

age in years)

To obtain your AMR from your BMR, multiply the BMR value by:

1.2 if you have a predominantly sedentary lifestyle (characterized by minimal or no physical activity)

A suitable alternative in a formal tone could be: A factor of 1.375 applies to individuals who engage in light physical activity, such as exercising 1-3 times a week.

A value of 1.55 applies if an individual engages in moderate activity, such as exercising or working at an average level.

If you engage in a high level of physical activity, such as rigorous training for six to seven days per week, your caloric intake should be approximately 1.725.

If you engage in frequent physical activity, such as performing strenuous physical labor or being a professional athlete, your activity factor is 1.9.

If you engage in minimal physical activity or do not exercise at all, you can be defined as having a sedentary lifestyle.

You can be characterized as moderately active if you engage in physical activity on a frequency of 1 to 3 occasions within a week.

You can be considered to have a moderate level of physical activity if you engage in regular exercise on a daily basis or if your occupation requires significant physical exertion.

You exhibit remarkable levels of activity if you engage in training sessions lasting over an hour for nearly every day of the week.

If one is engaged in manual labor or is a professional athlete, they can be considered exceptionally active.

Taking your AMR number into consideration, you possess all the necessary information to create uncomplicated and delectable meals, carefully portioned with the precise number of calories, alleviating concerns of an excessive conversion of ATP into adipose tissue or the depletion of muscle mass.

There exists a more convenient approach to adhere to your intended AMR without the necessity of meticulously tallying the caloric content of each individual component comprising a meal.

There exists a significantly more straightforward and convenient option. I merely compute the calorie count required to prepare a selection of my frequently consumed dishes.

I prefer to maintain a consistent dietary regimen and adhere to a meticulously calculated meal plan that accounts for the caloric content of every food item I consume. Therefore, I engage in the practice of combining and arranging ingredients according to the desired cumulative calorie content.

If I am aware of my intention to engage in a morning workout, I will consume a greater quantity of calories during the morning period. If I am aware of the fact that I will be experiencing a leisurely weekend, I opt to reduce my activities or commitments.

If comprehending the concept of BMR/AMR appears excessively complex, it is important to note that men typically expend approximately 2,500 calories, whereas women generally expend around 2,000 calories.

If you possess a physique that is considered average, it is advisable to create meals that maintain a cumulative daily calorie intake below either 2,500 or 2,000, depending on your particular somatotype.

Cherry Tomato Soup

- 1 tsp. dried parsley (or 1 tbsp. fresh)

- 1 tsp. dried basil (or 1 tbsp. fresh)

- 1 bay leaf

- 1/2 tsp. dried rosemary (or 1/2 tbsp. fresh, chopped fine)

- Salt and pepper to taste

- 1 cup chopped, red onions

- 3 large cloves garlic, chopped

- 1 tbsp. oil (I used coconut, but any oil you have will do.)

- 4 cups chicken broth, low sodium

- 1 lb. cherry tomatoes (I used red and yellow)

- 2 cups chopped broccoli

- 2 cups sliced baby carrots

Directions:

In a soup pot of medium size, set over moderate heat, proceed to sauté the onions and garlic in oil until the onions attain a translucent appearance. Stir regularly.

Effortlessly incorporate the chicken broth while introducing the tomatoes. Gradually raise the temperature until the mixture reaches a boiling point, and allow it to simmer for a duration of approximately 5-10 minutes, or until the tomatoes appear thoroughly cooked.

Now you have the desire to integrate or combine this. There are two available options: employing an immersion blender, preferably made of metal rather than plastic, or allowing it to reach a lower temperature before utilizing a blender instead. I employed my Vitamix blender to achieve a highly refined mixture. If employing a blender, kindly reintroduce the blended soup back into the pot.

Proceed to bring the soup to a vigorous boil, then incorporate all remaining ingredients with the exception of the salt and pepper. Incorporate this seasoning as per personal preference after the cooking process.

Please be sure to remove the bay leaf prior to consumption.

Paleo Egg Muffin Recipe

- 1 tsp Fresh Oregano (chopped or ½ t. dry oregano)
- 9 Eggs
- Dash of Pepper
- ¾ tsp Real Salt
- ¼ Cup Coconut Milk or Almond Milk
- 8 oz Pork Breakfast Sausage
- 1 Tbl Olive Oil
- ½ Sweet Onion (thinly sliced)
- ¾ Cup Bell Peppers (chopped or thinly sliced, any color)
- 1 1/2 Cups Spinach (packed)

Please ensure that the oven is preheated to a temperature of 350°F, and proceed to apply a layer of grease to the muffin tin.

Transfer the ground sausage to the pan and proceed to sauté it over a medium to high heat. Crush the pork using a spoon during the cooking process.

When it is partially cooked, incorporate 1 tablespoon. consisting of oregano, olive oil, peppers, and onions.

Cook the onion until it becomes transparent.

Next, incorporate the spinach into the mixture and carefully place a lid over the pan, allowing it to cook for a duration of 30 seconds.

Next, proceed to uncover the lid and thoroughly combine all of the ingredients. Remove from the heat.

Place the eggs into a sizable bowl, adding salt, milk, and pepper. Proceed to vigorously whisk the ingredients until the eggs have been thoroughly beaten.

Incorporate sausage and vegetables into the egg mixture and thoroughly blend.

Distribute the mixture equally among the oiled muffin tins, ensuring that each tin contains an equal portion (12 in total).

Place in a preheated oven and bake for a duration of 18 to 20 minutes.

Allow the contents to cool for a few minutes before removing them from the tins.

Grilled Chicken Panzanella

2 c. baby arugula

3 c. chopped watermelon, seedless

2 Tbsp. olive oil

¼ c. mint leaves, mints

1 tsp. honey

1 Tbsp. and 1 tsp. vinegar, red wine

2 oz. crumbled feta cheese

10 oz. chicken breast

Grape seed oil

½ tsp. paprika

1/8 tsp. salt

½ tsp. pepper

Cooking spray

½ sliced red onion

8 oz. whole grain bread, cubed

Directions:

Please activate the grill and proceed to raise the temperature. Apply a combination of pepper, salt, and paprika to season the chicken. Position the chicken upon the grill surface and allow it to cook for a duration of 15 minutes, until it attains an internal temperature of 165 degrees.

Remove the poultry from the grill and proceed to dice it into small fragments once it has cooled.

Set the temperature of the oven to 350 degrees. Apply a layer of cooking spray onto a baking sheet and place the bread on top. Transfer the bread to the oven and bake for a duration of 10 minutes to achieve a crisp, golden texture.

Whilst the mixture is in the oven, procure a bowl and blend a small quantity of pepper, mint, chicken, arugula, watermelon, and onion.

In a separate bowl, combine the honey, vinegar, and oil. Incorporate fifty percent of this dressing into the adjacent bowl and proceed to mix. Incorporate the bread and the remaining dressing into the mixture, ensuring they are evenly combined. Proceed to distribute the mixture into individual portions, then garnish with cheese prior to serving.

Spicy Miso And Pumpkin Soup

Ingredients

1/8 teaspoon white pepper

1 cup plain soymilk

3 tablespoons white miso

1/2 cup fresh basil leaf

Roasted soybeans, for garnish

1 tablespoon olive oil

1 medium yellow onion, chopped

2 garlic cloves, minced

1 (15 ounce) cans pumpkin puree

2 cups low sodium vegetable broth

1 cup water

1/8 teaspoon cayenne pepper

Directions

Sauté the garlic and onion in a pot with oil for a duration of 120 seconds.

Add in pumpkin puree. Add in broth. Add in water. Add in cayenne pepper. Add in white pepper.

Heat to boiling. Reduce the temperature and let it cook for a duration of 5 minutes.

Add in soy milk. Add in miso.

Please proceed to cook for the subsequent 60 seconds.

Transfer the soup to a blender and blend until it reaches a smooth consistency.

Incorporate the basil and blend for half a minute.

Incorporate the soy nuts as a topping.